CHAKRA HEALING FOR BEGINNERS:

A Beginners Guide to Balance Your Chakras for an Healthy Life Through Healing Meditation.

TABLE OF CONTENT

What Are Chakras?

Chakras are thought to be the overall centers of energy and spiritual power throughout the human body. We generally count 7 total chakras that go from the base of the spine throughout the entire body all the way up to the crown of the head. Each of these 7 chakras has a specific power and role and is believed to be what keeps us full of vibrant energy as we move through our lives.

Chakras can be thought of as constantly spinning wheels that serve to integrate our physical matter with our consciousness. Their invisible energy, known in as PRANA, is what we refer to as vital life force - the thing that keeps us healthy and alive. Science has found that Prana and the locations of the 7 major chakras in our bodies correspond with important nervous system junctions.

Each chakra is thought to be responsible for the proper function of a particular set of nerves, organs, and spiritual states of being.

Some people have even shown that chakras help the body maintain immune system function and regulate our organs day-to-day processes. Since the constant spinning motion that our 7 spiritual wheels are in is what helps our body systems function, it is important that nothing blocks their circular movement. Many people believe that the spiritual, mental, emotional, and physical problems we commonly experience are the result of damaged or blocked chakras. This book will help you learn more about how to tell if there is something wrong with your chakras and hopefully how to help you get them to return to proper function once again.

One important thing to keep in mind as you begin your research into chakras and how they function is that you yourself are a bundle of energy. All living things and everything you witness are comprised of energy. The chakras within help you regulate this energy and help your nervous system make conscious sense out of all these energies so that you can interpret your own soul and the world around you.

Chakras are also associated with their own colors and their own part of the body. Color visualization of the chakras in your body will help you distinguish between them and will help you isolate and balance damaged chakras.

History of Chakras

The idea of chakras stemmed from ancient Indian thought and made its first appearance in the oldest Sanskrit text called the VEDAS. Over the last century or so, Western Civilization has opened its arms and mind to yoga, and meditation from India, and has been uniquely captivated by the chakra system. However, since the majority of knowledge about chakras is in Sanskrit, an extinct language and the primary language of Hinduism, Western culture was slow to grasp the nuances of chakra health and the process of balancing energies within the body. So, as translation research began and more and more knowledge about the chakra ideology came out, chakras became more well known throughout the world. The entire chakra ideology is extremely complex and is still yet to be fully discovered. We will cover as much information as we can throughout the rest of this book.

In Sanskrit, the word chakra itself mean wheel, which is why we imagine the chakras in our bodies as spinning wheels or abundant and open flowers of energy. These energy vortexes have a history in Indian yoga philosophy, and so it is important to study chakras from their ideological source rather than Western adaptations of the idea. Chakras were originally meant to be a way for believers of Hinduism to get in touch with energies from their deities by repeating "mantras" in a type of prayer or meditation practice. Each chakra was associated with a particular deity or a particular element like Space, Earth, Fire, Wind, or Water. Hindus have a deep belief in their deities and in the world as a system - thus chakras were especially meaningful in ancient times because they were believed to be the one true connection between God and living beings. This system was extremely culturally and religiously specific, and so when it was adopted into Western cultures, some of this deeper meaning was eroded away. Today, the majority of people who are in touch with their chakras do not practice meditation for this purpose but do still receive benefits from the actions and balance. We will include some of these cultural and religious aspects, especially the concept of chakras relating to the world's elements, as we delve more into chakra practice. We will also make sure to include the more generalized Western school of thought on each topic we cover in this book. You will definitely have many choices with how you would like to think about your chakras and the way you would like to practice balance and meditation. In ancient India, chakras were introduced as an entire system throughout the body. Today, we refer to the 7 main chakras, an idea that became exceedingly popular among Western yogis around the 15th century. It is important to recognize that, although we will mostly cover this 7-chakra system in this book, the original belief puts various chakras systems all across the entire body and each system has a unique role in our lives. This might seem counterproductive because we are "ignoring" the rest of the chakra systems when we study our 7.

However, chakra ideology is not a fixed fact - instead, it is a fluid system through which you can discover your own primary energy supercenters. It doesn't matter which chakra-system you believe fits your body in the best way. History shows a variety of practices related to different chakras, but it is essential that you don't go into this feeling like one chakra system is better than another. You will certainly reap benefits from simply being in tune with your body's energy, regardless of which centers you tap into.

Type of Chakra

The Seven Main Chakras

To go through the seven main chakras is to do what you have just done in the visualization meditation. You can now "see" where they are and how they might look. They are "wheels" of energy along your spine, from tailbone to crown, and each has its own position of energetic power.

Each one may have its own unique qualities, however, they all work together as a team to support your energy overall. When you have blockages or imbalances, other energy wheels will compensate and either become to excessive in energy, or too deficient as a result. That is part of why it is so important to create the balance and clear the system of any wounds, pain, trauma, insecurities, fears, and repressed emotions.

When you are dealing with your own work on your chakras, you will have to be the judge of these "senses" or feelings about what you are not letting go of, or how you are projecting certain feelings through a certain chakra. This helps you to practice self-awareness so that you can be ready to gain more energetic life-force in your own system. It is a part of the healing journey to connect with yourself on every level and the chakra system can help you identify where you are the most blocked, uncomfortable and insecure.

The Root Chakra

Let's start at the base and work our way up, as you did in your visualization. The root chakra is located at the base of the spine is the color red. It has an energy of rootedness and groundedness and involves the quality of security and survival. It is your most basic and primitive need.

For many people, this chakra has the answers to all insecurities, doubts, fears and ancestral patterns that are repeated through the generations. It has a way of holding onto a lot of anxiety about wealth and financial security, as well as feelings of worthiness to have what you want and need to survive.

All of the energy of this chakra is very primal and supports the entire system when in a healthy flow and balanced vibration. It has the opportunity of awakening your kundalini energy, which is considered a more advanced form of chakra healing work that begins the whole-body alignment that leads to enlightenment.

Basically, this means that your root chakra is the beginning of soul awakening and the kundalini (ancient Sanskrit word to describe your coiled up, dormant life-force) is stored here until you are ready to "awaken" to your power.

The Sacral Chakra

Next in line up the spine is the second chakra. It is called the sacral chakra because it vibrates at the point of the spine where your sacrum is and has a lot to do with the energy of this area of your body. Inside of your body at this point is where a human being's sex organs are located. It is a part of us all to have passion and desire and that is the energy of this area.

When you think about the correlation to the placement, and the location of the uterus, ovaries and close proximity of the male gonads, then you can understand why this vibrational frequency would be associated with sexuality.

It is not all about sex in this chakra, however. There is the energy of creation, and not just of new life, like when you procreate to have children; it is about the creativity that exists in all life and everything that we do as people. We all have this creative energy and for some it is more productive and proactive than in others.

The sacral chakra is about creative life-force, as well as passion and desire. It has a great deal to do with our emotions and is connected to the element, Water. Emotions are watery and that is why there is a link to these energetic qualities. Many people assume that there is no need to have any creativity in their lives, or that they are simply not a creative person, when in reality, all of us is a creative life spark and sometimes a lack of creativity can come from an emotional block in the second chakra.

The Solar Plexus Chakra

Moving right on up the spine to the area just above your navel, we come to the solar plexus, or 3rd chakra, and it has a yellow color. Think of a bright sun glowing at this center of your body. It makes sense, since this chakra pertains to the element of Fire. This is the spot most commonly associated with the self and the power of "I am". It is an action-oriented center and has a lot to do with your personal power and how you achieve what you want in your life.

When you are happy in your life path and you are accomplishing all of your daily goals and life plans, this chakra is doing well and open energetically. It has a placement in your body that is all about energy. This is your vitality and strength. It is the location of where you digest food and convert it into energy for your whole body to use. It is how you work out your force and direct yourself forward in life.

There are a lot of possibilities for this chakra to become blocked, excessive, deficient or stagnant. Even though it is not numerically in the center of the chakra system, it is physically located between the upper and lower body. As you get into the heart chakra and move up through the crown, you are dealing with a different frequency of energies.

The Heart Chakra

Oh, the heart, the glorious heart. The 4th chakra is so named because of its location, just as with all of the other chakras, and is green in color. It has the position of being in the center of your chest as it is associated with the organ of love. Love is actually the energetic frequency of this chakra. While the sacral chakra is about passion and connection, the heart chakra is more about all forms of love, from platonic to romantic, to self-love and love for all humankind and the whole Universe. It is connected to the element of Air, just as love is whimsical and changeful.

The love chakra is about how you experience love, how you give it and how you receive it. It has everything to do with your compassion and empathy for yourself and for other people, too. When you are here, you know what it feels like to be hurt by love, to feel the intoxication of love, and to be overly giving of it, without receiving anything for it in return.

Most of us are looking for love and it has a very strong power. As we are all looking for it, we have also all likely been wounded by it at one point or another. This chakra is talking about how it feels to give what you want and ask for it in return. It is your right to know love in all its forms. To many people, it can be the most important quality of life and has been revered throughout the ages as the reason for living.

The Throat Chakra

Up into the neck and at the location where the throat meets the clavicles, is the 5th chakra. The throat chakra is a bluish hue and exists in the location of your voice. Not surprisingly, it is the chakra of communication and is connected to the element of Sound. Sound is how you breathe life into your self-expression and ask it to come forward in a language we can all understand.

The act of speaking brings the energy of your thoughts, feelings, power, passion and security in yourself into the world through the vibration of your vocal cords. No other chakra expresses itself the way that the throat chakra does and as such, it holds a special place in the system. The throat chakra is the communicator for all of the other chakras and brings the knowledge of each energy to the surface to be heard.

The Brow Chakra

Next in line along the chakra trail is the 6th chakra. The brow chakra is indigo and connects to the element of light. When you close your eyes and you picture something in your mind's eye, you can make out an image of light in this part of your mind. This energy center is commonly referred to as your third eye and it is the place where your sixth sense resides.

What is the sixth sense? This describes that part of every person connected to intuition, inner wisdom and even clairvoyance and psychic ability. Not all people believe that they have this kind of power, and yet the third eye would tell you otherwise. When your brow chakra has an ability to vibrate at its unblocked frequency, you can connect more to this aspect of yourself.

For a majority of people, there are significant blocks here and it can take years of energy healing work to become more enlightened and open in this part of the chakra system. People will often have beliefs and ideas that will confuse or distort their relationship to their "higher knowing", and so they may never truly become "awakened" in this energy center.

The Crown Chakra

Finally, at the very tippy top of your head is the 7th, and final of the main chakras. The crown chakra is violet and happens to exist as your gateway to connect to the divine. The placement of the crown chakra is very close to the brow and they are there together to create a connection to what many will refer to as "Source" energy. Source is not a religious energy or affiliation and is meant to describe the energy of all things in the Universe, and so we will not put a name on it, such as God, or Allah. It is whatever you believe in or practice. The crown chakra is where the Universal life force energy pours into you and allows for the transcendence of time, space, and human drama to become an enlightened being.

The crown is connected to the element of Thought. Thought is an energy, just as much as anything else, and our thoughts create realities. The journey to awakening your crown chakra takes time and has a lot to do with how you clear and rebalance your other, lower chakras. This is how you get to the point of feeling truly awakened to your total power and purpose so that you can live as a whole being.

The Science Behind Chakra

Moving forward with the chakras, there are even deeper ways to understand and explain the scientific reality of why they are there and how they can impact our body functions and mental states. The community of science relies upon the ability to measure something before it can be proven to exist. So, how do you measure a chakra inside of someone's body to prove that it is really functioning with all of the other systems?

In general, science and chakras are still shaking hands and getting to know each other, but there have been a lot of studies done in order to find ways to measure the presence of this energy. The energy frequency of certain vibrations is present in all matter and has given scientists a way to look beyond any religion, or esoteric belief, to have a more pragmatic approach to explaining chakras. There has also been the concept of biopsychology that allows understanding how the human mind, itself a giant electric center for productivity, compels the energy of the whole body to function, resulting in a balance between the energy centers of the body and the mainframe of the brain.

Vibrations and Frequency

Firstly, let's talk about vibration and frequency. Everything is made up of particles and those particles are throbbing life forms of energy. Everything about these particles has to do with the energy of how quickly or slowly they are vibrating. A vibratory speed is what will determine how a group of particles will form into a gas, solid, or liquid. It can be hard to imagine. You can't put your hand through your front door, even though it is just a bunch of particles vibrating together. In quantum physics, if you were to try and put your hand through your front door, the minuscule particles forming the door would become agitated, bouncing around and connecting to one another creating resistance. All of those throbbing, vibrating particles are a force field of energy, connecting to your energy and saying, "you shall not pass!"

A helpful way to try and picture this, or "feel" it, is to consider what is like when you try to put two magnets together when they are opposing particle forces. They will actually push each other apart quite forcefully. There is even a sense if you were to put your finger between the two opposing magnets, of an energy, or force field; a strong sense of their opposition to each other in the form of vibrating energy.

The invisible space between the two magnets which don't feel compelled to touch each other is made up of teeny tiny particles that work to stay in opposition, ensuring that there will never be a collision between the magnets. Vibrations of this nature cannot be seen by the naked eye and are therefore invisible. Remember those chakras? Chakras are made of energy as well and can have similar relationships with other energies in life or in the body.

Vibrations relate to this kind of energy, these swift and invisible particles that are holding up your desk chair, or the bus you are sitting on. The vibrations can be high or low, or somewhere in between. People will frequently say "good vibes" or "raise your vibes" as a way of stating, "change your frequency" or "increase your vibration."

Examples of emotions that might resonate at a higher frequency of vibration are compassion, kindness, hope, love and so forth. A low vibrating frequency is in the range of hatred, fear, dishonesty, and greediness.

People have done experiments to test these types of vibrational frequencies through using a tool, like a metal plate, that is connected to an amp or hertz frequency input apparatus. The plate is usually about the size of your average vinyl record, and kind of looks like one too. The plate is covered in sand and then, as the frequency of vibration is pumped into the metal plate, the sand will begin to vibrate as well and will change shape.

This technique, known as cymatics, is a great way to look at vibration in a physical way. There are plenty of online videos that you can look up to see the work of vibrational frequency in action to get a better idea of how it actually looks to see it happening.

The lower frequencies will create bigger shapes that are more distorted, and less intricate, while the higher vibrations will push the sand into something like to an intricate snowflake.

Taking this information, you can now apply the concept of vibrational frequency to the chakra systems. Studies have actually been done to prove that every chakra has its own frequency and that when we are out of balance it can mean that our vibration is what is imbalanced.

Chakra Frequencies

Chakra energy will sympathetically shift or alter in the company of other correlating frequencies, increasing the vibration to the point that it can actually be felt with our hands. Harmonic resonance is the term used to describe the sensation of feeling this energy.

Harmonic resonance will happen if there is a frequency, or vibrational wave, that connects to another object, presence of energy, or person attuned to the same energetic frequency, then causing a match in vibration. Examples of this are:

- Synchronized heartbeats between mother and child, or in a crowd of people

- Clocks ticking in tandem in a clock store

- Two instruments tuned to the same notes-pluck the string of one and witness the same string vibrate on the un-plucked instrument

Some researchers who have worked in the chakra system to uncover the science of frequencies have reported experiencing the impact of hearing or sensing a vibrational frequency alleged to be connected with a certain chakra. The root chakra, considered to be red, was paired with a color spectrum chart of vibrational frequencies that indicate that the color red falls somewhere between 430 and 480 hertz (hertz is the measurement of frequency). Testing out the spectrum of color frequency, the research team found that when they played a 432 Hz vibration, they could feel it resonate in their root chakras.

This evidence is so valuable and important as it gives a greater scientific link to the spiritual energy of our bodies. Having this kind of information helps us see that there is more to the body than just the cogs, wheels and moving parts and that our whole system is animated by the energy of vibrational frequency.

You could even think of your whole body as one, a great big musical instrument that needs continuous tuning with a tuning fork like you would tune a piano. As you think about tuning your instrument, imagine how the vibrational frequencies of every chakra are connected to each organ system and each emotional representation we might experience.

Biopsychology and the Chakras

Another aspect of the science of chakras is to talk about the mind -body connection and how they interface, or combine, through energy. Our minds are electrical computers that are always sending signals and messages to all parts of the body, and as that occurs, there are energy releases coming back into the mind from all of the energetic systems of the body. It's how we know when to react a certain way, protect ourselves, fight or flee, change our body mechanics to reflect our emotional state and so on.

The chakras in our body system work as centers of an organization to transmit, integrate, receive and transport all of our life force energies. The elements that you read about for each chakra, from root to crown are earth (root), water (sacral), fire (solar plexus), air (heart), sound (throat), light (brow), and thought (crown) play a significant part in our whole system integration from the mind center. These "energies", or elements of life, are what bring our capacity for wholeness into flow and resonance.

As we study the structure of our physical bodies through anatomy and physiology, we study the concept of the soul and the psychology of how we react and respond to life, through our mind and emotions. All of this is bridged by the vibration of the chakras and their ability to help us effectively handle the life force of our energy. The programming we receive throughout our lives has a great impact on our ability to flow freely through our energetic wholeness.

Throughout your life as a person, you grow up dealing with life's ups and downs, trials and tribulations, childhood wounds and woes, and all of the aftermath, defenses and beliefs about ourselves that might accrue as a result of the path we walk and the people who show up on it. All of these psychological, emotional and physical experiences can get stuck in the form of energy in our chakras and as we get older, we may not even realize that these blocks exist.

From the standpoint of what you have already learned about vibrational frequency and the chakras, your overall vibration can resonate at a certain frequency your whole life without you even realizing what the cause of it was in the first place. It would be like discovering that your G string has been out of tune on your guitar since you were eleven and you just thought that that is what a 'G' note was always supposed to sound like.

From the point of view of psychology and the understanding of vibrational frequencies, you can see how a lifetime of certain "vibrations" could cause you to feel blocked, unhappy, isolated, or various other feelings. The associations of certain emotional and psychological realities to certain chakras help you identify another angle of how to heal a past wound or emotional block that you haven't fully let go of. Sometimes, therapy isn't enough, and you need another mode of healing.

Using biopsychology as a way to promote another kind of healing, empowers your energy centers to clear and flow more smoothly. The processes of breaking through a psychological perspective, pattern, behavior or belief, through understanding the qualities of the chakras and their vibrations, is another unique way to explore the science behind how we are attuned as beings, not just of thought and physical matter, but energy, frequency, and colorful light.

All of the research on chakras comes from years of practicing from the perspective of healing and growth, and yet in today's modern society, and with the technology of our time, scientists and researchers are spending more time trying to find out what it is that truly makes us feel, function and thrive. Deciding to look beyond the spirituality and more deeply into the physics and psychology of how chakras work can really help you notice that beyond our sight, there is an actual throbbing energetic field that has always existed in and around us.

Myths About Chakras

As with anything else in the world, myths get created when people don't take the time to learn about new things. There are myths circulating about chakras, which are the energy centers that run many parts of your physiology. This will include your physiological, psychological, and emotional tendencies along with your organs. Chakras help to determine the well-being of a person.

You need to be aware of all the truths and myths about chakras before actually trying to balance or open them.

There aren't any chakras.

There are many stories that claim chakras don't exist. There are a lot of people who refuse to even acknowledge their existence. But there are many places in the world that have their own meanings and proof that chakras do exist. The seven chakras symbolize the nerve or energy centers that are present inside every human body. Energy or Prana flows throughout the body through nadis. These are three channels similar to electric cables that take energy from the electricity center and supply this energy to the entire body. The three channels, or nadis, are Ida, Pingala, and Sushumna.

Opening chakras is easy.

You may find a whole bunch of literature out there about how you can open your chakras to heal yourself and get rid of any troubles you might be having in life. It might be emotional or physical problems among others. The truth about awakening your chakras isn't as easy as books say it is. Opening your chakras requires a shift and change in consciousness. This requires many years of meditation. You can't just open your chakras by doing yoga poses, and it isn't an emotional process.

Having the chakras balanced will definitely improve health.

This misconception is huge. Balancing the chakras *can* improve your health. How healthy your chakras are, all depends on your psychological, physiological, emotional, mental, and physical conditions. If you don't work on these problems, your chakras won't shift and change, and your conditions won't ever improve.

Chakras have to be perfect and balanced at all times.

If you have heard anyone say that chakras have to be perfect and balanced all the time, they are living in their own little world. In the real world, nothing is perfect, and every single thing has imperfections. Our world is unpredictable and changes constantly and this is how chakras behave. They are constantly changing, too. They are responsive and flexible. Chakras adjust to physical and psychological factors that affect us daily.

They change as your current emotional and physical states change. They have to be normalized and balanced to deal with the current situation.

Professional healers can balance and open your chakras in one session.

Most people like to turn to professional healers like Acupressurists and Reiki healers to try and heal and balance the chakras in one sitting. This is a huge myth that is circling the globe. It will always take more than one sitting and more help than a professional healer to open and balance your chakras. It takes YOU wanting to be healed in order to do it.

You need to take charge of your emotions and body in order to be healed. You can get the help of professionals to heal your chakras, but it is up to you, not them, to heal you.

There are seven chakras.

Many theories say there are only seven chakras in our body. In the Yogic text, there are many chakra systems throughout the body. Some believe there are as many as 12 chakras; others think there are more systems that work in the body. Beginners are taught and told about the most common seven chakras.

Chakras are just "things" that live in our bodies.

Everyone should know that chakras aren't material things. Some people might not have thought about what this really means. We speak as if an autopsy will show a string of different colored lotuses going through the center of our torso. Possible thinking suggests that a chakra is another organ such as the spleen or liver. Chakras are major energy channels on a plane of consciousness that results in psychosomatic functions and experiences. They serve as focal points for spirituality and meditation. Here are some definitions:

- _Intentionally based abstract structures

- Visualization in a yogic body

- Spinning consciousness in our bodies

The main purpose of chakras is to treat illness.

If you look at ancient Vedic literature, chakras refer to wheels and are the seven centers in the body. If opened, they can unfold to unforeseen realms that have been a main goal for many people who want to be one with the Universe.

Most of what people do today to balance and open their chakras is used to treat emotional pain and physical illnesses. It doesn't deal with the consciousness and awareness of our Supreme Self.

This is what has happened to yoga in our modern world. Yoga is often seen as nothing more than gymnastics, and doing a few asanas means you are now a yogi. The ultimate goal for yoga is meant to meet the Divine Source or our Supreme Consciousness by attaining the Samadhi through meditating. This has been forgotten and the true purpose and goal for yoga have been totally blinded.

You can't control your chakras.

Many people think you don't have any power over your chakras and you can't balance them by yourself. The truth in the old saying, "Where there is a will, there is a way" holds true with controlling your chakras. The solar plexus chakra can help strengthen your inner desire, fire, and will. It doesn't matter what problems you are dealing with, you can harness this power and reach any goal you want to accomplish. This is true for every chakra in your body. They give you energy for many different tasks.

You should only worry about the top chakras.

Often people only want to worry about the top chakras which are the throat, third eye, and crown chakra. These are responsible for inner and spiritual growth. People forget they have to be balanced from the lower ones to the top for the body and chakras to work together.

The heart chakra is responsible for balancing the bottom and top chakras. Before trying to work on the third eye and crown chakra, you need to work on the lower ones.

The root chakra symbolizes our physical life. The sacral chakra symbolizes our emotional center. The solar plexus symbolizes our power center. If you want to be successful in life, you need to work on balancing your chakras from the bottom to the top. Begin at the root chakra. After you have worked on your emotional and physical problems and gotten them disciplined, you are ready to focus on your main purpose in life. Now, you are ready to balance the top chakras.

Healers can remove all your problems and Karmic baggage.

There is a law of cause and effect that is active in this Universe. This law is responsible for everything that goes on in the world. Thinking that all of our actions – from this and previous lifetimes – and Karma can be handled by someone in just a few sessions, it is so completely wrong.

The intensity of your Karma can be reduced, and you can increase your willpower when you balance your Karma, but all the baggage can't be removed by anyone in healing sessions.

We have to think about these points before we move toward the path of balancing our chakras.

Chakras are energy sources.

Visualize a whirlpool. A whirlpool isn't just motionless water but a vortex of water. This same principle applies to chakras. They aren't sources of energy, they are places where energy moves and gathers. Chakras are balls of spinning energy that are three dimensional and absorb and emit energy from the world. To balance and heal our chakras, we have to call on outside sources such as pure Spirit energy, grounding earth energy, or channeling Reiki energy.

What is the correct way to pronounce "chakra" in its most original form?

Do you remember learning this tongue twister when you were young: "How much wood could a woodchuck chuck if a woodchuck could chuck wood?" Now repeat, "chuck, chuck, chuck". Now add "ra" and you got it — "chuck-ra". In the official translation convention for Sanskrit, the "c" gets pronounced as "ch" as in "church". You might see "cakra" and "chakra". It doesn't matter how one spells it, just remember woodchuck.

The sacral chakra is about sex.

There are a lot of desires that can play out through karma and instinct. We have a natural desire to gain freedom and experience, to express ourselves, and to live. Instead of thinking about certain desires as exclusive to certain chakras, you need to think about desire as a natural state of humans and the foundation of life. Remember that every school of yoga supports mastery, transmutation, or transcendence of sensual desires even though they might differ in the way the transcendence takes place.

The Benefits of The Different Chakras

So far, we've mostly been looking at the chakras as a system. But it's important to go back and look at all the ways in which each chakra is different as well. Though they all work in harmony to regulate your energy, each chakra has a number of different attributes that it's good to remember when learning about chakra healing.

Root Chakra

The important thing to remember about the Root Chakra is that it grounds your energy in the earth and the material world. It is the base of the ladder that the rest of the expansive chakra system is built on.

No other chakra is this related to the material world. It is a very instinctual chakra, mainly concerned with food, self-preservation, sex, and sleep.

If you're looking to find more stability in your life, this is the chakra to focus on. It allows you to make good decisions, stay organized, and act with common sense.

There are a number of scenarios in which focusing on the Root Chakra would be beneficial. For example, perhaps you may have trouble budgeting month-to-month. You find yourself spending too much money, more than you can afford, or racking up debt for things you don't need. This, no doubt, leads to stress and a decrease in your energy levels.

There could be a number of causes for this. However, it's worth exploring how an imbalanced Root Chakra could be causing this. It could be that your Root Chakra is blocked, causing you to not be grounded enough when it comes to financial matters. In that case, you would want to meditate and do other healing actions to unblock this chakra, focusing on how it grounds you to your financial realities. By meditating and contemplating this, you may find it easier to take more responsibility when it comes to budgeting, easing the stress this causes.

On the other hand, you may find that you are having trouble letting possessions go, and that you may be participating in hoarding behaviors. This could be driving a wedge between you and those around you, especially your loved ones.

This could be caused by an overactive Root Chakra, causing you to put too much value on your material possessions. Here, meditation and contemplation will help you understand the proper balance of both your chakra's energy and your attachment to the material world.

Sacral Chakra

The Sacral Chakra applies to number of situations in your life, being much more tied into your body's emotional needs. This is where the energy for satisfying your needs for human identity, emotion, and creativity is kept. This will help you in scenarios that have to do with your emotions and desires, deciding whether you will control them or be controlled.

When you are enjoying life through the senses and your emotions, this chakra is responsible. It is this chakra that allows you to maintain a balance between appreciating the pleasurable things in life and overindulging. It also is the well-spring for your creativity, allowing you to respond and adapt to changing circumstances and fueling your creative passions.

A scenario in which focusing on this chakra may be beneficial is if you are having problems achieving sexual pleasure. If you are experiencing problems in your sex life, such as impotence, a blocked Sacral Chakra may be responsible.

It could be, of course, that another chakra is responsible for restricting the energy flow to this area. It is important to meditate to see how your chakras are blocked, and how they may be interfering with your energy flow. It could be that something is causing you to feel an inability to achieve pleasure in all aspects of your life, not just your love life. In that case, unblocking the Sacral Chakra will help immensely.

Conversely, if you are too focused on sex, giving into fantasies and not practicing balance and moderation when it comes to your sex life, it could be that your Sacral Chakra is overactive. In that case, balancing it is the imperative thing to do.

Navel Chakra

Remember that in this chakra is our personal power, the force of will that drives us forward in our lives and gives us momentum. This chakra provides you with a sense of self-confidence and empowerment, serving to hone honing your personal power to go through your life with confidence, determination and strength.

This chakra provides you with power and momentum to keep moving forward. It gives you the willpower to take your ambitions and intentions and make them a reality. It also is in charge of your direction in life, and can influence your self-perception.

When the Navel Chakra is balanced, you'll feel confident, steadfast, and empowered in your decisions and in the direction of your life. This helps you be in balance with your relationships with others. It also makes things happen so that you'll feel a greater sense of purpose in your life, beginning to understand who you are and why you are here, and you'll begin to let go of the material things that you have begun to overvalue.

However, when this chakra is out of balance, you may begin to feel weak, guilty, or experience low self-esteem. If this chakra is deficient or blocked, you may begin to feel less assured in yourself, experience feelings of helplessness and irresponsibility, and have trouble making decisions. This can hinder your ability for self-expression, or lead you to make plans without realizing efficient ways to execute them. If this chakra is overactive, however, you may feel angry and ill-tempered, aggressive or controlling.

For example, if you find that you want to switch careers, but you can't build up the momentum from with to move forward and make this change happen through the force of your will, it may be that you have a blockage in this chakra. In this case, it would be good to meditate on this and understand what the forces are that are blocking your Navel Chakra, and what is causing this stress in your life.

On the other hand, for example, you may find that you are frequently talking over people around you, and not letting anyone else get a word in. This could be because the Navel Chakra is putting too much power into your will and self-confidence. In this case, you'll need to reduce this chakra's energy output to bring it into balance and not put strain on your personal relationships.

Heart Chakra

This chakra provides you with love, compassion, and kindness, both to give and receive. Centered on the heart, this chakra is based around these highly positive aspects, promoting love for others as well as love for yourself. It also helps you tap into a sense of unconditional love, as well as connecting you to other properties of the higher self.

The heart chakra is the bridge between Earth and Heaven, between the more earthly chakras and the more spiritual ones. This chakra is also associated with healing, aiding you with transformation and change and helping you grieve and reach peace.

once you have the Heart Chakra balanced, you'll be able to choose compassion and love, even in situations where it's difficult. You'll be a loving person, sharing compassion with yourself and others equally. A balanced Heart Chakra will allow you to feel connected with the world around you, and give you a deep appreciation of beauty.

However, when the Heart Chakra is imbalanced, you may feel difficulties relating to others or even to your own emotions. If this chakra is overactive, you may put others too far before yourself and sacrifice too much of your own well-being for the love of another. If this chakra is blocked or underactive, however, you may feel cut off from emotions, making it hard to relate, empathize, or connect with family, friends, and those around you.

For example, if you are feeling that you can no longer empathize with what your close family is going through you may have a blocked Heart Chakra. Any method that would boost this energy would most likely help you in this situation.

Alternately, you may come to realize that you are always trying to make your friends happy, to the point that you don't have enough energy to care for yourself. In this case, your Heart Chakra is probably overactive. Through meditation and contemplation you can learn to dial it down and balance out your loving energy.

Throat Chakra

This chakra is highly focused on your personal voice and your ability to express yourself. It is this chakra that provides the energy that helps you project your ideas and your truth into the world.

The energy of the Throat Chakra is not only tied to speaking truth, however. It is also deeply connected to your ability to live a life in accordance with your values and beliefs. It is this chakra that provides you with the ability for clear communication and conviction.

when the Throat Chakra is in balance, you'll feel confident to share your inner truth and wisdom, enlightening and enriching the lives of those around you. You'll feel outgoing and able to connect with others. You'll also feel a sense of purpose and validation in your chosen path.

However, when this chakra is no longer balanced, you may begin to have issues with your communication. If your chakra is overactive, you may talk over others and keep others from sharing their truth. It could also lead to you talking too much, or being aggressive and mean in your interpersonal conversations. A blocked Throat Chakra may leave you feeling timid and unable to express your thoughts around others. It can lead to introversion and a sense of insecurity.

For example, you may find that you have a hard time standing up to people when your viewpoint on life is different from theirs. You may feel that you don't have the courage or conviction to make that happen. In that case, your Throat Chakra may be blocked. Unblocking this would provide you with the energy you need to state your truth.

As another example, you may find that others are reluctant to speak around you, because you come off as overbearing. In this case, an overactive Throat Chakra is to blame. Keeping that energy in check will help you navigate your relationships much more easily.

Third Eye Chakra

This very important chakra is the door to the spiritual world. It provides you with intuition and allows you to gain knowledge that you would otherwise never be able to reach.

This chakra gives you the ability to perceive energy beyond the physical world, achieving a connection with higher planes of existence and higher levels of consciousness.

When not serving as that sort of door, this chakra is associated with inner knowledge and self-assurance. It not only allows you greater insight into the world around you but also to yourself.

An example could be if you don't feel that you have a vision for where you are going, or what you want to accomplish. You may feel that you don't understand who you are well enough to commit to a path. In this case, meditation on the Third Eye Chakra can help.

Crown Chakra

The Crown Chakra is what allows you to connect your consciousness to the consciousness of the entire universe. This chakra allows you to transcend your physical self and commune with the divine. With access to this chakra, you understand wisdom and all else that is sacred. It allows you to commune with higher states of consciousness, leaving behind the boundaries of space and time.

It is possible that through this chakra you will feel a sense of union with the universe – a very beautiful sense of bliss. Clarity and wisdom come easy to you during this state.

Therefore, instead of seeing how an imbalance in this chakra is negatively affecting your life, you should strive to understand all the positive and sacred implications that opening up this chakra can have.

Bringing A Balance In Life

When we are doing anything with our chakras, we are playing with higher energies. These are energies which can easily go out of our control if we are not careful enough. You can never take these energies lightly.

Bringing a balance in your life is even more important than bringing a balance in your energies. If your life is not balanced, any area where you are trying to provide more energy can become overactive. The process of balancing also requires clearing denser energies from some parts of your body. Even that energy is not going anywhere.

First of all, you will have to understand the real meaning of energies flowing in your body. The energy in your root chakra and the energy in your crown chakra are not different in their form. They are exactly the same. It is the kind of use where it is utilized. It is exactly like air. The same air is present all around you; you know it is important but never feel its presence. When you are blowing your hair with a hairdryer, you feel that air as it is being thrown at a greater speed. The same air starts looking dangerous when it is part of a storm. The form of that air changes when it is coming out of the propellers of a jet. It is not the air that changes in all these events. It is the current source and how it manifests that air.

So the dark energy excessive in one chakra will eventually be used to balance the others. It is the same life energy flowing in your whole body. If your life is not balanced, it will not be able to use energy in a proper way.

Like water takes the shape container where it is placed, the energies will also try to find the areas they can take over. So if you are not balanced internally, the energies will keep messing with one chakra after another. If you don't want to fall into the vicious cycle of continuous maintenance, you must remain balanced and focused. The biggest threat is from the energies around you. When you start clearing your chakras, the darker energies present around you will also try to gain access. You simply become a more receptive body of energy. If you are not balanced and determined, you can develop fears and phobias. The best way to avoid such problems is to adopt some methods to balance your life.

The Vedic methodology is all about correcting the ways of life. It helps you in improving your karma. People have started wrongly associating Vedas with religion, specifically, Hinduism, Buddhism, and Jainism. As per the Vedas, there is no such religion as Hinduism. It is called 'Sanatan Dharma.' It means an eternal way of life to be followed by humankind. It lays down principles for a meaningful life for every individual.

It gives great importance to certain principles of maintaining sanctity in life. Those principles are as follows.

Mindfulness

You must always remain mindful in life. When you are mindful about your actions, you tend to generate the lowest amount of negative karma. When we take actions without giving much thought about them, we tend to hurt a lot of people and other creatures. That would increase the negative influence of energies on us. We will have to fear more. We will have to be more careful; we will have to be more conscious. All this takes away the peace from life. It weakens our energy system. Our energies get channeled in the wrong direction.

When you practice mindfulness, you the grounded in the present. You are more aware of your surroundings and the consequences of your actions. This prepares you better to fight the negative influence of dark energies.

Gratefulness

This is one of the most important things to practice to increase the influence of positive energy inside you. When you practice gratuity, you leave no place for the influence of negative energies inside you. Your body fills with positive energy, and the darker energies present outside are not able to take over you. The influence of darker energies and thoughts is the highest when you are filled with negativity about others. There is a sense that you didn't receive what was due to you. Unknowingly, you open yourself up for negative energies. On the contrary, when you are grateful, you are more in a giving mode. The influence of positive energies is higher; hence, the negative energies around you are not able to make headway.

When you practice chakra awakening, balancing, and healing, there is bound to be an interaction with a lot of energies. It is a part of the process. It is important that you prepare yourself for the process physically, mentally, as well as emotionally.

The more sweetness you have inside you, the lowest will be the impact of negative energies, influences, and emotions. Even if the energies in some of the chakras increase, your sweetness of emotions will simply accentuate positivity; hence, you will be able to balance the energies in due course of time.

The best way out is to practice gratefulness for everything around you. The easiest way to do that is to lower your expectations from others and invite pleasantness.

An Active Life

Chakra balancing means drawing out energies from some chakras where they are aggressive and sending them to the areas that are energy deficient. This happens best when you are active. If you can do meditation, yoga, qi gong, or other physical activities, it would be best for you. However, even walking, exercising, and similar physical activity is also good as it helps in the proper movement of energy inside you. A sedentary lifestyle makes the energies stagnant, and the process of opening up of chakras becomes tedious.

Even if you have a busy schedule, try to walk as much as possible. Yoga is one of the best ways to channel energy inside your body. Physical activity also helps in warding off the influence of negative energies present outside.

Consecrated Spaces

This is a bit difficult part for many people to understand. They feel that they can try to meditate anywhere and get the same results. If they prey anywhere, it will have the same impact. This is a misunderstanding.

We all have energies. We are a big pool of energy besides the physical mass of blood and bones. When we pray or meditate at a particular place, we are leaving a part of our positive energy at that place. If we continue to pray or meditate at the same place regularly, we will increase the positive energy of that place. This will make focusing on meditation much easier. You would find that you are able to reach the meditative state easily. You will get disturbed by thoughts much less. You will fear much less as the influence of positive energies is higher.

The same goes for religious places. It is the reason some religious places have greater significance than others. The simple reason for that is the higher accumulation of positive energies at those places.

Therefore, it is important that you pick a particular spot in your home for chakra activation, healing, and balancing. If you want to meditate, that place would be the best for the purpose. If you want to pray, that place will provide you the greatest peace. The only reason for that is clearing out of negative influences. The more time you spend there, the higher will be the influence of positive energies at that place.

Shuddhi or Purification

Purification has a very important role in the pranic system. It says that if a place is not cleared of the negative influences, it will keep disturbing you. Before you designate a place for such purposes, it is important that you clear out that place of all kinds of negative energies.

The most effective way to do this is to meditate and do chakra awakening in a separate room. Such rooms should be free of all physical things that are not required. Even pieces of old furniture that are not essential should be removed from such rooms. The room should be as minimalist as possible. This will ensure that things that can have any kind of negative influence or may cause distractions are absent.

However, if that's not possible due to space constraints, the specific place chosen for chakra activation should be free of excessive things. You must keep that place very clean and maintain the sanctity of that place. Generally, separate rooms are advised as the approach of other people can be limited to those rooms. If you cannot find such a room, you should try to limit the access of other people to this room as much as possible. Every person has energy influences, and the exchange of energies is a continuous process. If people with negative energies are moving in and out of such rooms frequently, they will keep disturbing the energy levels of your room. This will make the process of chakra activation and balancing difficult and time-consuming.

You can also use incense sticks, candles, and other such objects to bring positive energy into the place. Maintaining the energy balance and increasing the influence of positive energies is the most important. The biggest problem with having negative energy in your room would be difficulties in building focus. If the influence of negative energies is higher, you will keep getting disturbed and distracted.

Epsom Salt Baths

If you are a person who comes in the influence of negative energies very easily or someone who has a delicate energy balance, you must consider Epsom salt baths. Epsom bath salts are really beneficial in warding off negative influences. They are also very helpful in case you suffer from physical aches and muscular troubles.

The specific benefits of Epsom Salt Baths are as follows.

It helps in relaxing your body as well as your mind. The magnesium in the salt helps in relaxing your muscles that make you feel relieved. If you have racing thoughts, then this bath can help as it relaxes your mind and triggers it to slow down.

If you are having sleep disorders, this bath can help you greatly in sleeping well. The magnesium in the salt nourishes your neurotransmitters.

The sulfur content in the salt also helps in detoxification of the toxic elements received from the environment.

Your digestion would also improve considerably as it stimulates the production of certain enzymes in your gut that aid digestion.

It helps in relieving anxiety. You'd feel more secure and at peace.

Epsom salt baths help in clearing your auric field. It means that you don't take the influence of other people's energy center. If you come in contact with a person who has a strong auric field, it would not affect the energy balance in your body. This is a big problem when you are actually trying to balance energies in your body because the balances are delicate at that point. Your body becomes more receptive to influences. In such situations, you should take Epsom salt baths at regular intervals.

Epsom salt bath also helps you in remaining grounded. The sulfur in the Epsom salt is a major foundational stone that provides an amazing grounding effect. Irrespective of the chakra you are trying to balance, proper grounding is essential.

How to Heal You Chakras

How to Heal Broken Chakras

It is not difficult to learn how to repair your own chakras, be it through holistic medicine, crystals or whatever method works best for you.

Root Chakra

Fear, worry, and uncertainty weaken this chakra the most—and the quickest. In order to regain courage and the drive to accomplish your goals to move further in life, here are some things you can do:

1) Give someone a hug, or ask someone to give you a hug.

2) Give yourself a back rub for about 15 minutes.

3) Raise a plant at home to keep you more connected with earth and nature, two very important methods of survival and success. Another way to keep in touch with nature is to go for a walk, barefooted.

4) Plan an outdoor picnic.

Sacral Chakra

Feelings of guilt are not good for a healthy sacral chakra. Here's what you can do to help fight that off:

1) Go get yourself a massage to loosen any stiffness and tightness you have in your body. This physical improvement will also help you improve emotionally.

2) Use aromatherapy or Epsom salts when you take a bath. These products help get rid of negative energies.

3) Do something with art to keep your creativity flowing.

4) Get into baking, as it is actually relaxing and therapeutic for both your mind and hands.

5) Write love notes and poetry.

6) Get rid of dirt and all the unwanted clutter in your home. Those are a distraction and deter you from accomplishing what you have planned for the day.

7) Show love and positivity not only to yourself but also to others.

Solar Plexus Chakra

If you find yourself reacting to any kind of traumatic, troubling event--especially when the event is unexpected—in a mature, calm manner, especially when you react overemotionally, then you know that your navel chakra is weakened. Here are some solutions to help you learn from these events and move on:

1) If someone is directly mean or nasty towards you, fold your hands over your solar plexus to block the negative energy from them.

2) It is natural and perfectly fine to outwardly express your anger, but is never okay to take it out on others in harmful ways, physically or verbally. Instead, do something more constructive by writing, drawing or punching a soft object, such as a pillow.

Heart Chakra

If you ever feel unable to love, or that you love someone so much you become bitter and jealous, you need to repair your heart chakra, using some of these guidelines:

1) Think of some of the positive qualities in a person that you admire, but also remember to focus on the positive attributes of yourself instead of being self-deprecative. At the same time, don't let your self-admiration devolve into egotism and conceit. You must also be aware of your flaws and how to fix them.

2) Surround yourself with people who respect and encourage your positive spiritual growth. These people don't necessarily have to share the exact same spiritual beliefs as you, but they should be able to help you and help you grow, especially during times of need.

3) Do some yoga and stretching.

4) Get in touch with nature as much as possible.

5) Count your blessings and remember all the good things that happened in your life.

6) Write a list of wishes for yourself, and hopefully, they are realistic enough to be fulfilled one day.

Throat Chakra

Keep your throat chakra healthy and functioning by being honest with others and yourself. Also, keep your creativity awake and get inspired if you feel yourself suffering any kind of creative block:

1) Plan what good things you will do for others each day, even if it's a simple compliment or gesture of kindness.

2) Go an entire day without complaints and take criticism with a grain of salt, no matter how harsh.

3) Sing a song. It's a good release of and from tension.

4) Let external surroundings, such as noises from nature, guide you and aid in your creativity.

5) Listen to any and all good advice others have for you.

6) When someone says something mean or horrible to you, completely ignore them.

Third Eye Chakra

Again, the only way to keep your third eye chakra healthy is to be sure to not let your imaginations deter you from having a grip on reality. Here are ways in which you can do that:

1) Look at beautiful artwork and/or watch a beautiful, uplifting film.

2) Plant yourself a meditation garden, with whatever vegetables, fruits and other plants you love most.

3) Decorate your home with uplifting, positive quotes or pictures.

Crown Chakra

No matter how spiritually inclined of a person you are, you must never forget that you're still human like everyone else. In order to acknowledge that so that you maintain your willingness and desire to keep growing as a person, as a delusion of perfection, in addition to a sheltered existence, means no real growth and learning.

1) Reflect on events, both good and bad, of your past and don't let them define you but rather use them as lessons to improve and enrich your life, and to be grateful for all the good things that happen in your life.

2) Keep your spiritual connection and relationship with whatever Deity it is you choose to worship.

3) Be charitable, but not for the praise. Do it because it's TRULY from your heart.

Different Methods to Heal Your Chakras

You don't need a psychic to help you repair your damaged chakras. You can do it yourself! There are easy techniques to do so, and you have a lot of alternative remedies to choose from if one of the techniques does not work.

First Chakra

The biggest challenge for the root chakra is fear—so you need to develop courage, and realize that you're meant for bigger and better things. For that, you could use these affirmations below:

1. Hug someone, or ask someone to embrace you. This helps you become more grounded.

2. Rub your lower back for about 15 minutes. Do the same with your buttocks.

3. Lie in a very comfortable bed. A comfortable sleeping place will renew your energy.

4. Keep a plant in your home and take care of it. The soil will make you connect with Mother Earth.

5. Cook your favorite meals.

6. Begin your day with dancing.

7. Take a walk, preferably barefoot. It's a good grounding practice. It will take away any stress that you feel.

8. Have a picnic.

9. Recite mantras or affirmations with the following terms: health, security, responsibility, honesty, fairness, routine, organization, work, order, flexibility, and honesty.

10. Your power statements are "I need, I want."

11. Say any of the following statements.

Second Chakra

Being your body's passion and pleasure center, the main challenge here will be guilt, which can only be combated by taking risks—and by believing in yourself. Here's what you should do:

1. Get a good and relaxing massage. Reflexology will help loosen up the knots that you feel, not just physically but also emotionally.

2. Practice aromatherapy. Whether you are using candles or incense sticks, take time to smell the natural essences, and let them fill your lungs with renewed vitality.

3. Take sensual baths with Epsom salts. This kind of salt cleanses away the negative energy around you, purifying your chakra points.

4. Eat chocolate. Chocolate is an anti-depressant and is rich in antioxidants.

5. Work with clay or wood. Get your hands working with nature's best art resources.

6. Get a good haircut and feel good about yourself.

7. Feel the vibrations around you. Attune yourself to the sounds and sights, to the secret messages of the universe. Feel the

connection between you and the soil, you and the flowers. Feel the energy coming from your fingertips. Put your hands over your crystals and feel the warm energy pouring forth from your palms.

8. Bake bread. Kneading distracts the mind and the heart, and the smell of pastry is good for you.

9. Take care of plants in your house. Bring nature to your indoors.

10. Relax in a rocking chair.

11. Write love poems and write love notes to someone.

12. Clean your house to get rid of negative and unwanted vibes.

13. Spread love and cheer to other people. The good energy will bounce back to yourself.

14. Say a mantra with the following terms: passion, love, vitality, desire, comfort, pleasure, beauty, sexuality, and indulgence.

15.Say the following affirmations.

Third Chakra

The main challenge that the Solar Plexus Chakra faces is how you can be aware of your personal power, and how you'll be able to use it in a way that's balanced and fair. In short, you have to be consciously responsible, and you have to be able to react to the circumstances in your life in the right way.

To do that, it's best that you do the following:

1. Protect your solar plexus chakra by folding your hands over it when someone angry is speaking to you. Doing so blocks the negative energy coming from that person.

2. Pretend to be someone you dislike so much so that you will know what it is like to be in their shoes. You don't have to go overboard; just knowing how they feel is enough.

3. Express your anger. You can write, punch a bean bag, cry or scream in the shower. Use whatever method of catharsis is available to release your pent-up emotions.

4. Act in the theater. Channel someone else's personality. Be other people for one day.

5. Throw a costume party at your house or be a cosplayer.

6. Know what your mission in life is. This will give more depth to you as an individual. You will become more aware of your purpose, and all your actions will have direction.

7. Your affirmations should be about focus, commitment, dedication, faith, choice, courage, discipline, autonomy, willingness, cooperation, and authority, examples of which are as follows.

Fourth Chakra

The Heart Chakra is able to move through your life. It's able to help you get in touch with yourself and appreciate life better—and that's why its biggest challenge is grief. You then have to use affirmations to improve this chakra, and so you could live your life to the fullest!

1. Be someone's secret admirer. It doesn't have to be the romantic kind. You could admire someone for the way they talk, dance, cook, or write. Learn to appreciate the talents of others.

2. Write yourself a love letter. What do you want to tell your sixteen-year-old self? Write that down, including admonitions and inspirational messages.

3. Apologize. Acknowledge your faults and shortcomings.

4. Build a spiritual family. This family will help you through rough times, especially when you need help in taking care of your spiritual needs. Your spiritual family could consist of

your relatives, friends, colleagues or people from your church.

5. Look at your baby picture. Remember that you have an inner child. Don't strive to be a perfectionist.

6. Adopt a pet. This is good for the soul because you learn to take care of others.

7. Stretch on the bed, or do yoga.

8. Connect with nature. Take care of plants in your house. Put your hands under running water. Stand in the shower for several minutes as you relax your mind.

9. Create a gratitude list. Thank the universe and God for giving you your desires.

10. Create an altar. Put whatever you feel is important to you and always pray at that altar.

11. Create a "desires box". This is where you put all your wishes and desires. Write them on a piece of paper and do your best to achieve them within a year. Turn them over to the

universe and believe in the power of the universe to grant your wishes.

12. Say the following affirmations.

Fifth Chakra

Throat Chakra is one of the most spiritual chakras. This inspires you to be creative and expressive—as well as being honest with yourself. Its main challenge are lies—you have to be able to see through them and, at the same time, make sure that lies will not rule your life.

1. Have a good and positive motto. For example, Today, I will speak kind words to people. The good chi that you feel will also be channeled towards other people.

2. Think that something positive will happen every day. Don't expect bad things to happen.

3. Breathe deeply and listen to a variety of sounds. Close your eyes and hear the sounds of the birds chirping, the cars passing by, the neighbors chatting.

4. Avoid complaining for one whole day and accept any criticism thrown at you.

5. Sing. This beats those unwanted energies. You will instantly feel good, too.

6. Learn a new language. It doesn't matter if it's French, Spanish, or Japanese. It's cool to learn another set of cultures and symbols.

7. Let go of the past. Let go of the emotional baggage that holds you back. Wear a black obsidian gemstone if you have to.

8. Practice saying things in advance, especially when you think you don't feel comfortable in a situation.

9. Empower yourself with the mantra "I am." Complete the statement with any adjective you want to say. You could say, "I am strong. I am powerful."

10. Take a chance. Give people the opportunity to speak to you. Grab opportunities for change, too.

11. Keep yourself from retorting. It only brings bad vibes.

12. Then, don't forget to utter the following affirmations.

Sixth Chakra

The Third Eye Chakra is also spiritual in the sense that you can appreciate both your inner and outer worlds. Your main challenge here is an illusion. You have to know how to blur the lines between reality and fiction; you have to learn to live in the real world, while still being able to use your imagination.

1. Watch good and beautiful films.

2. Look at a beautiful work of art, or place one at home or on your working desk.

3. Create your own greeting cards.

4. Place a bowl of fresh fruits near you.

5. Have a professional photo of you taken at the studio of your choice.

6. Create a mood board and visualize all the dreams and ambitions that you have in life.

7. Have a meditation garden. Plant/place all of your chosen plants and flowers here. Go here if you are troubled or if you want to meditate.

8. Attach magnets or any inspiring notes and photos on your fridge.

9. Train yourself to see auras. Relax and adjust your eyes until you see a colored halo above the head of another person. Do this often and you will begin to see auras in no time.

10. Your affirmations should contain the following words: invention, memory, clairvoyance, daydreams, insight, visualization, and open-mindedness. For this, you could try the following affirmations below.

Seventh Chakra

You have the crown chakra, which helps you become selfless and unite with every part of your body. Its biggest challenge is an attachment. You have to see things as passing things—as things that just come and go in life, the way most people do.

This way, it will be easy for you to accept change—and understand that it's really the only constant thing in life. Here are the affirmations you could use:

1. Compose a story about your past life. It could be funny, serious or scary. You will notice some similar points in your life until you

realize that that same story explains your very fears and your personality.

2. Listen to classical and Baroque music.

3. Cancel out all the negative energy from the food you eat, or from the objects you hold.

4. Rest on Sundays.

5. Talk to the Higher Being, whether it is God, or Allah, or the Nature Goddess.

6. Allow the sound of a bell or a chime to resonate in your body and in your home.

7. Be a philanthropist and help the needy without asking for anything in return.

Healing Meditation

Chakra meditation is a simple and highly effective way to bring balance into your life, and energize your chakra centers. This chapter will be dedicated to familiarizing you with a chakra meditation that is simple and easy and that will benefit you mentally and physically. You will need willpower and a level of devotion when performing this meditation to fully reap its benefits.

Preparation

It is important to prepare where you will be doing your meditation. You can actually do this anywhere, but you will need a quiet and peaceful area. Choose a place and time when you will most likely not be distracted. Choose a spot you are comfortable in too. You need to be relaxed for this to work after all. You can get a meditation pillow to help you keep your posture straight.

Things to remember:

- This meditation technique will take about half an hour, so make sure that you will not be disturbed during that period.

- Choose a position you are comfortable in. You can lie down or sit on a chair, or you can choose to take on the lotus position.

Get in a comfortable position that you can hold on to for 30 minutes. Close your eyes and take long deep breaths. Be aware of your breathing and keep it controlled. Remember to maintain a gentle focus rather than a forced one. Feel your body relax with every breath. If you find it hard to get relaxed, you can try to do some stretches beforehand or say some affirmations to yourself, such as, "I am calm, I am relaxed."

Visualization Meditation

Start centering your focus on the crown chakra, the chakra found at the top of your head. Visualize white light flowing in through your crown chakra and into the body, filling you with warmth and energizing you. Feel your fears, guilt, anger and all your negative emotions being washed away in a shower of light. Notice that your thoughts are clearing away as well, which leaves your mind clear and calm. You will soon notice that your crown chakra is full and the energy has stopped flowing. It is now time to transfer that energy toward the brow, or third eye chakra.

Feel the energy flowing down from your crown, which is now a bright purple color, to your third eye chakra, glowing and filling up the vortex with light. Visualize the brow chakra a light with bright purplish blue color. You will know that the energy from the crown has lowered toward the third eye chakra once you feel the energy flow stopping. Now visualize the energy flowing down to the throat, this time with the throat chakra glowing a vibrant blue.

Visualize and feel the warmth flowing, from your throat chakra to your heart, from your heart to your solar plexus and so forth until you reach your root or base chakra. Remember the corresponding colors of the chakras (green for the heart chakra, yellow for the solar plexus, orange for the sacral chakra and red for the root chakra). If you happen to have a certain illness in that part of the body, such as headaches (brow Chakra) or digestive problems (Navel chakra), envision the illness as a dark speck that slowly disappears in the light of the cosmic energy now coursing through your body.

If you feel like a center chakra center of yours is weak or has low energy, you can visualize your chakra as having a dull color, or a different color than what it is supposed to have. Envision it becoming the color that it's supposed to be as the white energy flows down into that chakra.

You can't expect this meditation technique to work if there is doubt in your mind. You have to really give yourself to the meditation and dispel any expectations before you go into it. If this is your first attempt at meditation, you may or may not feel something. Don't get disappointed or frustrated. It takes patience and continued practice to finally open up your chakras.

Guided Meditation

In many ways, meditation can be like a prayer. It's an intimate process that everyone approaches differently. On the other hand, through the years it has been discovered that certain meditation techniques offer unique advantages. How you approach meditation will impact the results you achieve. With that in mind, it's worth looking at how guided meditation can help you make the most of every minute you spend in meditation.

The idea of guided meditation is that the person meditating is following the instructions of a guide. It comes from the many traditions where experienced spiritual leaders would pass on their knowledge by guiding their students in the spiritual arts that they had discovered. The unique thing about guided meditation in the modern era is that now students don't have to go out and meet masters, they can listen to meditation instructions from just about anywhere.

It helps to know the best meditation techniques. If you understand basic principles and kundalini techniques, you will be much better prepared. A little bit of knowledge can go a long way, whether you're looking for someone to guide you, a pre-recorded message to follow, or a personal plan for meditation.

The value of mantras

One of the things that set kundalini meditation apart from other approaches is the use of mantras. Rhythmically chanting while meditating is a powerful way to improve the results of your meditation.

The importance of breathing

Another thing to look for in kundalini meditation is breathing. Regulating the flow of breath is one way that we can master our bodies and reshape the way we feel, act, and think. If this sounds extreme to you, just try to practice serious breath control and you will soon feel the power yourself.

As with mantras, there is no one pattern for breathing. Different breathing patterns can be used to bring about different results. You can change how much air you breathe in, how quickly you exhale, and how you alternate between exhaling and inhaling. That's right, you don't have to stick with breathing in and breathing out. You can also chain together multiple inhales but switching to multiple exhales. This can help take your mind to some really interesting places.

The importance of pacing

Kundalini meditation is not for people who need constant action. It's about intentionality, not speed. It takes time to activate your chakras one by one. This isn't something you can turn on like you're flipping a light switch. It is a gradual and methodical process.

This doesn't mean that you have to commit to long and drawn-out meditation sessions. You can start with short sessions and add on more time as you go along. But even if you are only meditating for five minutes, you still need to be slow and deliberate if you want to unlock full kundalini potential. Your energies take time to wake up. The only way to speed up the process is to do it consistently so that your energies aren't allowed to fall too far out of balance.

The value of visualizations

Another common element of truly effective meditation is visualization. It can be hard to wrap your head around some of the things we talk about because we are discussing forces that are invisible to the naked eye. This is why we use visualization to give some form to the thoughts we are dealing with.

Some visualizations are very abstract, helping to convey emotions or the flow of energy. Others are more literal, asking you to picture a certain scene within your mind. Different teachers use different approaches.

The importance of energy

There are many ways to approach meditation. Each has its own value, but any system that doesn't center on our spiritual energy misses the mark by at least a bit. Any program of guided meditation that isn't designed to work with the natural flow of energy won't give you everything you need.

This isn't to say that you can't attend a less spiritual meditation workshop and privately focus on your own spiritual energies. Still, this goes against the principle of guided meditation. Suddenly you are deviating from the directions of the teacher, which is not something that encourages a healthy learning environment. So, understand that it is possible, but it's better to use a meditation routine that is explicitly designed to work with your spiritual energy.

Finding Guidance

It's easy to see why guided meditation is a good idea, but it can be harder to find the right person to guide you. As we said earlier, meditation is an intimate exercise, and it isn't always easy to find someone whose approach meets your needs.

The good news is that in the modern era it's easier than ever to find the guidance you seek. If you go online, you'll find plenty of resources where you can find recordings where gurus will lead you through a session of meditation. Still, there's no replacement for dealing with people in person. Life is about the flow of energy that connects all living things. You might find that meditating as part of a larger group helps you to achieve a new level of balance while raising your vibration levels.

Remember that while you look for guidance, it helps to seek out individuals who share your spiritual focus. The fact of the matter is that while meditation and yoga were both created to deal with our spiritual energies, many people only see the physical results they produce. People who aren't interested in the spiritual may feel the change brought about by meditation, but they don't understand what truly causes it.

While you should never judge anyone for believing differently than you do, it can be helpful to find someone who is on a similar spiritual path. This is especially true when seeking out someone who can provide you with guidance. You don't want to find yourself in a situation where the blind are leading the blind.

If you can ask the person who will lead the meditation about things like chakras and kundalini and get a meaningful response, then they might be someone to listen to. You don't have to know about such things to discover the fundamental truths behind meditation, but it certainly helps.

The most effective guided meditation

So, after all is said and done, you might be wondering what you should do. There are so many options to choose from, of course you'd want to know which is the best.

The honest answer is the best option is the one that inspires you to continue meditating. That's why there's no perfect option. Everyone is different.

The full value of meditation is only unlocked once you develop a habit for meditating. If you like to take a certain class or listen to a certain online guru, then follow your inspiration. As long as they aren't leading you in toxic directions you will find that the time spent in silent reflection will help you put things into perspective.

You should never get so caught up in chasing perfection that you never commit to anything. Find what works for you and stick to it. That's the road to success.

Self-Examination

As someone becomes more in tune with their chakras and learns how to maintain and keep them open, this regular maintenance is not the end of their expanded consciousness—it is just the beginning. Because even with finely tuned chakras there is still much to be learned. In this chapter we will examine just how you can take things further, once you get beyond the initial seven chakras.

Higher Dimensional Chakras

As you become better in tune with your chakras, your whole spiritual "frequency" will eventually find itself being broadcast in a higher dimensional plane. Here the colors and the hue of the chakra—for those clairvoyant enough to see them—are said to become rather distinct, and the energy circuits begin to flow much quicker. This is the most evident over the "heart chakra".

For those that have reached this higher dimensional state, with the influx of positive energy they feel, they can be said to be quite literally "open hearted", with brilliant, positive light flowing forth from their heart chakra. At this stage of chakric development, the individual is said to begin to have a whole new outlook on their fellow man, and begin treating others with true compassion, understanding, and brotherly (or sisterly) love at all times.

Prana and the Breath of Life

In yogic teaching the simple act of breathing is connected with the power circuits of the human chakras. The act of breathing in and out is connected to "prana" which is the "primordial impulse" that motivates all functionality of living breathing creatures. Prana is the spark of life that keeps us all going. It is for this reason that tradition teaches that the ability to monitor and maintain our own influx of prana can lead to a much healthier body and mind.

It is for this reason that breathing exercises are so important when it comes to meditation and other yogic practice. Breathing involves the process of many aspects of living. It connects you directly to the physical atmosphere that you are breathing in oxygen from, to your physical organs of respiration, and ultimately every oxygenated tissue of your physical form. Breathing is also the only aspect of your "autonomic nervous system" that we are normally able to actively control.

But breathing as it turns out is the gateway to harnessing sway over the rest of your automated bodily function. Because there are trained yogic masters who have perfected their breath of life to such an extent that they are reportedly able to do things such as lower and raise their blood pressure at will, and even actively control how fast their heart beats. All of this all thanks to a better understanding of prana and the breath of life.

When we are fully conscious and fully aware of our breathing and our surroundings, there is a constant communication taking place between our individual concept of self and the "extended" perception of self that connects the individual with the larger environment. Just consider the molecules that go through your lungs on a daily basis that also pass through the physical forms of other living creatures all over the planet and perhaps all over the entire universe as well.

If one considers this undeniable fact, all living breathing creatures do indeed appear to be linked—if not by anything else—by the fact that we breathe the same air. The same molecules that went through a polar bear, an elephant, and yes even a cockroach, will eventually be recycled back into the atmosphere and go through yours as well. Under the ancient tradition, this is nothing short of your personal "chakric energy" combining with the energy of the universe at large.

The Science of the Chakras

As scientific studies in the realm of physics—especially in regard to quantum mechanics—continue to advance, there has been much scientific data that has amassed which seem to corroborate much of the chakric teaching. For one thing, it has been well established that there are indeed energetic particles invisible to the naked eye, in fact these particles surround us on a daily basis. Wherever we may go—we may not see them—but they are there nonetheless.

If you are the beneficiary of internet Wi-Fi for example, consider the fact that whatever device you may be using is being bombarded with a steady stream of invisible molecules in order to give you a constant stream of the internet. You cannot see or detect the signals being put out, but they are there nonetheless sending out a constant stream of data to your device. The truth is, there are a countless number of electro-magnetic waves and particles being sent in your direction at all times.

Whether it be from radio, TV, cellphones, or as mentioned, from the internet—these invisible waves of energy are there. We know that these dense packets of information being beamed at us exist because when we turn on our TV, switch on a radio, or attempt to use Wi-Fi, we will receive some sort of input for our efforts. Chakras and the electromagnetic waves that emanate from the human body are just as real, even though they too are invisible to the eyes of most.

What is the Eighth Chakra?

Although basic chakra teaching is an overview of just 7 main chakras, according to tradition there are more. There is in fact, an eighth chakra which is considered the conduit for all "divine love" and "spiritual compassion". It is said that this is also the chakra that contains all of our "karmic residue". According to traditional belief, this is the place where your previous longstanding emotions reside, whether in this lifetime—or as some believe—across previous lifetimes.

If this 8th chakra petal is allowed to bloom, it opens up the individual great "spiritual awareness", and unity among a true "community of beings". This chakra is also said to be the "gateway" for "spiritual perception", and even "astral projection". Most have not fully developed their eighth chakra, but once they do they will see an immediate difference in their life.

How do the Chakras Relate to Acupuncture?

Acupuncture is an ancient Chinese tradition that involves the manipulation of certain points on the body in order to effect change in physical conditions. These points are not all connected to a chakra but many of them are. There are many teachings that seek to combine and join the understanding of the energetic chakras with that of the more physical acupuncture points.

In fact, in an effort to bring these two systems together there are some that have developed the so-called "chakra points" in which the energetic flow of the chakra is used to complement the physical points of acupuncture. These combined therapies typically begin with the crown chakra and work their way down. The therapy is then carried out through the use of typical acupuncture needles placed into the acupuncture locations. During the process the acupuncture patient is guided into focusing on the chakra point that corresponds with the needles that are being inserted into them.

Although the jury is still out on just how effective such a practice may be, there are many who would give a glowing report, and tell us that there is nothing better than the combination of these two ancient practices. If you feel compelled to take such a treatment, keep an open but cautious mind. And if find that your health problems become unmanageable even through the use of chakras and acupuncture, you should seek the immediate help of your doctor.

Sensing the Chakras by Touch

If someone would like proof that such a thing as chakras exist, all they really have to do is reach out and touch them. There are minor chakra points located in the palms of your hands for example, and they are perhaps the easiest to sense. Anyone can detect these points of energy by engaging in a simple yogic exercise. Simply hold your palms slightly apart as if you are praying, and hold this pose.

Keep the palms separated by just an inch or so and focus on the energy radiating from between your palms. At first you may not feel anything right away, but with time you will begin to notice the flow of energy from one palm to the other. Similarly, the other main chakras can be perceived as well. The heart chakra for instance can be felt simply by placing your hand in the middle of your chest, near where your actual physical heart resides.

You will obviously feel the warm rush of blood, and perhaps the beating of your physical heart, but you will also begin to sense a steady crackling of energy flowing through this important conduit. So too, can all of the main chakras of the body be felt, and experienced through touch. It just takes a little time and practice, but anyone can learn to directly sense their chakras in this fashion.

Once you are used to the process, this is actually a great means of monitoring and checking up on the status of your chakras. Those who are knowledgeable of such things are able to gauge how well their chakras are performing at any given time simply by touch. If you are ever doubtful of just how well your chakras are performing, the simple sense of touch can tell you much.

Is the Practice of Chakras Compatible with other Religions?

Although there has been much confusion and debate over whether or not belief in chakras constitutes a belief in religion, the truth is that the chakras at face value are just a discovered set of energy points said to be flowing through the body and nothing more. Although the findings of such energy points are crucial in empowering the mind and body, it is not of any more significance than discovering the brain, lungs, heart, or any other organ of the body.

Just because you know where your kidney is located and how the kidney functions does not mean that you are suddenly some fanatic adherent of a kidney-based religion, it simply means that you know how this very important organ functions. In that sense, the practice of chakras should be compatible with any given religion. For Christians for example, there is nothing in the Bible that discusses chakras one way or the other. From the Christian perspective, as long as you are not attaching chakra belief to any other deity, it should not pose a problem for Christian belief.

Conclusion

Understanding ourselves as a human being is crucial in enabling us to deal with issues affecting us in our daily lives. The Chakra system does more than just helping us with our problems and goes further to enable us to have a good health and even deal with future situations or difficulties.

Using the available techniques to keep our chakras open is very important. It will help you deal with a serene and full life. You will also be able to maintain excellent relationships, develop knowledge, connect with the universe, and even connect with our spiritual being.

We have also learned the best way to learn the techniques of opening your chakras is by practicing them more regularly, creating awareness and focus while opening, healing, or balancing the chakras. When our chakra system is functioning properly, our lives are organized and all-inclusive. Also, meditating, exercising, and practicing yoga as regular as possible is generally a good idea if we wish to maintain balanced chakras and a good quality of life.

Chakras also help us with getting more integrated and feel wholeness with our lives and gain confidence that we might not have discovered we are capable of displaying when dealing with our challenges.

The book has extensively covered the topic of the chakras system and numerous ways in which it can be organized to enhance the quality of life. Besides visualization and various approaches discussed to help gain enhanced quality of life, another vital thing is the help an individual discovers hidden potential which he/she can activate, utilize and gain greater fulfillment in his/her life.

Lightning Source UK Ltd.
Milton Keynes UK
UKHW012305290721
388013UK00001B/169